EAT TO BEAT CROHN'S DISEASE

Crohn's Disease Cookbook: Recipes And Symptom Management Techniques

DR. LONDYN DELANEY

Copyright © 2024 By Dr. Londyn Delaney

All Rights Reserved...

Table of Contents

Introductory 5

CHAPTER ONE 10

   Importance Of Diet In Managing Crohn's Disease 10

   Goals Of A Crohn's-Friendly Diet 16

CHAPTER TWO 23

   Foods To Avoid & Foods To Include 23

   Common Nutritional Deficiencies In Crohn's Disease & Solutions 31

CHAPTER THREE 40

   Diet During Flares & Diet During Remission 40

   Post-Surgery Diet 50

CHAPTER FOUR 58

   Steps To Implement An Elimination Diet 58

   Meal Planning For Crohn's Disease 65

CHAPTER FIVE 73

   Recipes For Easy Digestion 73

   7-Day Sample Meal Plan For Remission 83

CHAPTER SIX 93

   7-Day Sample Meal Plan For Flare-Ups 93

Breakfast, Lunch, And Dinner Recipes......102

Dinner Recipes 108

CHAPTER SEVEN..114

Snack And Smoothie Recipes 114

Smoothie Recipes 116

Specific Carbohydrate Diet (SCD) For Crohn's Disease..121

Gluten-Free Diet For Crohn's Disease 127

Low-FODMAP Diet For Crohn's Disease....133

Vegan And Vegetarian Diets For Crohn's Disease..141

CHAPTER EIGHT..149

Lifestyle And Dietary Strategies For Long-Term Management 149

Common Questions About Crohn's And Diet 156

Summary...161

THE END...164

Introductory

Inflammation of the intestines and colon is a hallmark of Crohn's disease, a kind of inflammatory bowel disease (IBD). The ileum and the beginning of the colon are the most typical sites of infection, although it can affect any portion of the GI tract (from the mouth to the anus). Several symptoms and problems might develop as a result of the inflammation that Crohn's disease causes.

Symptoms

Common symptoms of Crohn's disease include:

- Diarrhea
- Abdominal pain and cramping
- Fatigue
- Weight loss
- Fever
- Reduced appetite
- Blood in the stool

Causes:

The exact cause of Crohn's disease is unknown, but several factors are believed to contribute to its development:

- **Immune system**: An abnormal immune response may cause the immune system to attack cells in the digestive tract.
- **Genetics**: Crohn's disease tends to run in families, suggesting a genetic component.
- **Environmental factors**: Certain factors, such as smoking, diet, and stress, may increase the risk of developing the disease or trigger flare-ups.

Complications:

Crohn's disease can lead to several complications, including:

- Bowel obstruction
- Ulcers
- Fistulas
- Anal fissures
- Malnutrition
- Colon cancer

Diagnosis:

Diagnosis of Crohn's disease typically involves a combination of tests and procedures, including:

- Blood tests
- Stool tests
- Colonoscopy
- Endoscopy
- Imaging tests (CT scan, MRI)

Treatment:

There is no cure for Crohn's disease, but treatment can help manage symptoms and induce remission. Treatment options include:

- Medications (anti-inflammatory drugs, immune system suppressors, antibiotics, etc.)
- Nutritional therapy
- Surgery (in severe cases)
- Lifestyle changes (diet modifications, stress management, quitting smoking)

Management:

Managing Crohn's disease often involves a combination of medical treatment and lifestyle adjustments. Regular monitoring by healthcare professionals and adherence to prescribed treatments are crucial for controlling symptoms and preventing complications.

CHAPTER ONE
Importance Of Diet In Managing Crohn's Disease

Diet plays a crucial role in managing Crohn's disease, as it can help control symptoms, promote healing, and maintain overall health. While there is no one-size-fits-all diet for Crohn's disease, certain dietary strategies and modifications can be beneficial for individuals with this condition.

Importance of Diet in Managing Crohn's Disease:

Symptom Control:

• **Identifying Trigger Foods**: Some foods can exacerbate symptoms like diarrhea, cramping, and bloating. Common trigger foods include high-fiber foods, dairy products, fatty or fried foods, spicy foods, and caffeine. Identifying and avoiding these foods can help reduce flare-ups.

- **Low-Residue Diet**: During flare-ups, a low-residue or low-fiber diet can help reduce bowel movements and ease symptoms. This diet limits high-fiber foods such as whole grains, nuts, seeds, raw fruits, and vegetables.

Nutritional Balance:

- **Preventing Malnutrition**: Crohn's disease can lead to poor absorption of nutrients, resulting in deficiencies. A balanced diet that includes a variety of nutrient-rich foods can help prevent malnutrition. In some cases, nutritional supplements may be necessary to ensure adequate intake of vitamins and minerals, such as vitamin B12, vitamin D, iron, calcium, and folic acid.

- **High-Calorie, High-Protein Diet**: During periods of active disease or recovery, individuals may require a diet high in calories and protein to maintain weight and support healing.

Reducing Inflammation:

- **Anti-Inflammatory Foods**: Incorporating anti-inflammatory foods such as fatty fish (rich in omega-3 fatty acids), fruits, vegetables, and whole grains can help reduce inflammation in the digestive tract.

Maintaining Hydration:

- **Staying Hydrated**: Diarrhea and malabsorption can lead to dehydration. Drinking plenty of fluids, especially water, is essential. Oral rehydration solutions can also help replace lost electrolytes.

Individualized Diet Plans:

- **Personalized Nutrition Plans**: Working with a registered dietitian or nutritionist can help create a personalized diet plan tailored to individual needs and preferences. This can include meal planning, identifying safe foods, and managing food intolerances.

Managing Specific Complications:

• **Strictures and Fistulas**: In cases of strictures (narrowing of the intestines) or fistulas (abnormal connections between organs), a modified diet that includes soft, easy-to-digest foods can help prevent complications and discomfort.

Practical Tips for Managing Diet in Crohn's Disease:

- **Keep a Food Diary**: Track food intake and symptoms to identify potential trigger foods.
- **Eat Smaller, Frequent Meals**: Smaller, more frequent meals can be easier on the digestive system.
- **Cook and Prepare Foods Carefully**: Opt for cooking methods that are gentle on the digestive tract, such as steaming, boiling, or baking.

- **Stay Informed**: Stay updated on new research and dietary recommendations for Crohn's disease.

While diet alone cannot cure Crohn's disease, it is a vital component of managing the condition. A well-planned diet can help control symptoms, promote nutritional balance, reduce inflammation, and improve the overall quality of life for individuals with Crohn's disease. Working closely with healthcare providers, including dietitians and nutritionists, is essential for developing an effective dietary strategy tailored to individual needs.

Goals Of A Crohn's-Friendly Diet

A Crohn's-friendly diet aims to achieve several key goals to help manage the symptoms and complications of Crohn's disease, promote healing, and maintain overall health. Here are the primary goals:

1. Symptom Management

Reduce Inflammation and Alleviate Symptoms:

- **Identify and Avoid Trigger Foods**: Foods that commonly exacerbate symptoms include dairy products, high-fiber foods, fatty foods, spicy foods, and caffeine.

- **Low-Residue/Low-Fiber Diet**: During flare-ups, this diet can help reduce bowel movements and alleviate symptoms like diarrhea and abdominal pain.

2. Nutritional Adequacy

Ensure Adequate Nutrient Intake:

• **Balanced Diet**: Include a variety of nutrient-rich foods to prevent deficiencies.

• **Supplements**: In cases of malabsorption or specific nutrient deficiencies, supplements may be necessary (e.g., vitamin B12, vitamin D, iron, calcium).

3. Weight Maintenance and Energy

Maintain Healthy Weight and Energy Levels:

• **High-Calorie, High-Protein Diet**: Especially important during flare-ups or recovery periods to prevent weight loss and promote healing.

4. Hydration

Maintain Adequate Hydration:

- **Fluid Intake**: Ensure sufficient fluid intake to prevent dehydration, particularly during bouts of diarrhea.

- **Oral Rehydration Solutions**: Use these to replace lost electrolytes if necessary.

5. Reduce Digestive Stress

Minimize Stress on the Digestive System:

- **Small, Frequent Meals**: Eating smaller, more frequent meals can be easier on the digestive system than large meals.

- **Soft, Easily Digestible Foods**: During flare-ups or when dealing with complications like strictures, choose foods that are easy to digest.

6. Anti-Inflammatory Benefits

Incorporate Anti-Inflammatory Foods:

- **Omega-3 Fatty Acids**: Found in fatty fish (such as salmon and mackerel) and flaxseeds.

- **Fruits and Vegetables**: Choose those that are less likely to cause irritation, and consider cooking them to make them easier to digest.

7. Individualization

Tailor the Diet to Individual Needs:

- **Personalized Diet Plans**: Work with a dietitian to create a diet plan tailored to individual symptoms, preferences, and nutritional needs.

- **Monitor and Adjust**: Keep a food diary to track symptoms and adjust the diet accordingly.

Practical Tips for a Crohn's-Friendly Diet:

- **Food Diary**: Keep track of food intake and symptoms to identify patterns and trigger foods.

- **Cooking Methods**: Opt for gentle cooking methods like steaming, boiling, or baking rather than frying or grilling.

- **Probiotics and Prebiotics**: Incorporate these to support gut health, if tolerated.

- **Avoid Problematic Foods**: Common culprits include dairy (for those who are lactose intolerant), high-fiber foods (during flare-ups), and highly processed foods.

A Crohn's-friendly diet is tailored to manage and minimize symptoms, ensure nutritional adequacy, maintain hydration, and reduce digestive stress. It is a personalized approach that adapts to the individual needs and responses of those with Crohn's disease, with the ultimate goal of improving quality of life and overall health. Working closely with healthcare providers, including dietitians, can help create an effective dietary plan that addresses these goals.

CHAPTER TWO
Foods To Avoid & Foods To Include

Managing Crohn's disease effectively often involves making careful dietary choices. Certain foods can exacerbate symptoms, while others can help manage and alleviate them. Here is a guide to foods to avoid and foods to include in a Crohn's-friendly diet:

Foods to Avoid:

High-Fiber Foods (during flare-ups):

- Whole grains (e.g., whole wheat bread, brown rice)
- Nuts and seeds
- Raw fruits and vegetables, especially those with skins or seeds

Dairy Products:

- Milk, cheese, ice cream, and other dairy products (if lactose intolerant)

Fatty and Fried Foods:

- Fried foods (e.g., french fries, fried chicken)
- High-fat meats (e.g., bacon, sausage)
- Heavy cream and butter

Spicy Foods:

- Hot peppers
- Spicy sauces and seasonings

Caffeinated Beverages:

- Coffee
- Tea
- Energy drinks

Carbonated Beverages:

- Soda
- Sparkling water

Alcohol:

- Beer

- Wine
- Spirits

Sugary Foods:

- Candy
- Cakes and pastries
- Sugary cereals

High-Fiber Legumes:

- Beans
- Lentils
- Chickpeas

Certain Raw Vegetables:

- Broccoli
- Cauliflower
- Brussels sprouts
- Foods to Include

Low-Fiber Foods *(during flare-ups):*

- White bread

- White rice
- Refined cereals (e.g., Cream of Wheat)

Lean Proteins:

- Chicken breast
- Turkey
- Fish (especially fatty fish like salmon and mackerel)
- Tofu

Cooked Vegetables:

- Carrots
- Peppers
- Squash (well-cooked)
- Potatoes (peeled)

Fruits:

- Bananas
- Applesauce
- Melons

- Canned fruits (without added sugar)

Low-Fat Dairy Alternatives:

- Lactose-free milk
- Yogurt (if tolerated, especially probiotic varieties)
- Plant-based milks (e.g., almond milk, soy milk)

Grains:

- Oatmeal (if well-tolerated)
- Rice cereals
- Quinoa (if tolerated)

Healthy Fats:

- Olive oil
- Avocado (in moderation)
- Flaxseed oil

Hydration:

- Water

- Herbal teas (e.g., chamomile, peppermint)
- Broths (clear, low-fat)

Additional Tips:

• **Probiotics and Prebiotics**: These can help maintain gut health. Yogurt with live cultures and fermented foods like sauerkraut may be beneficial if tolerated.

• **Small, Frequent Meals**: Eating smaller, more frequent meals can help ease digestion.

• **Cooked and Pureed Foods**: These are often easier to digest and can reduce the risk of irritation.

• **Hydration**: Drink plenty of fluids, particularly water, to stay hydrated.

Creating a Crohn's-friendly diet involves avoiding foods that can trigger symptoms and including foods that are easier to digest and provide necessary nutrients.

It's essential to tailor these recommendations to individual tolerances and work with a healthcare provider, such as a dietitian, to develop a personalized eating plan. Keeping a food diary can also help identify specific foods that may cause flare-ups and those that help manage symptoms.

Common Nutritional Deficiencies In Crohn's Disease & Solutions

Individuals with Crohn's disease often face nutritional deficiencies due to malabsorption, inflammation, and sometimes due to dietary restrictions during flare-ups. Here are some common nutritional deficiencies associated with Crohn's disease and their solutions:

Common Nutritional Deficiencies and Solutions:

Vitamin B12:

- **Cause**: Malabsorption, especially if the terminal ileum is affected or has been surgically removed.
- **Symptoms**: Fatigue, weakness, anemia, neurological issues.

Solutions:

- **Dietary Sources**: Animal products such as meat, fish, dairy, and eggs.

- **Supplements**: Oral B12 supplements or intramuscular B12 injections.

Iron:

- **Cause**: Chronic intestinal bleeding, poor absorption due to inflammation.
- **Symptoms**: Anemia, fatigue, weakness, pallor.

Solutions:

- **Dietary Sources**: Lean meats, fish, poultry, fortified cereals, legumes.
- **Supplements**: Oral iron supplements or intravenous iron infusions in severe cases.

Vitamin D:

- **Cause**: Malabsorption, limited sun exposure, dietary restrictions.
- **Symptoms**: Bone pain, muscle weakness, increased risk of fractures.

Solutions:

- **Dietary Sources**: Fatty fish, fortified dairy products, egg yolks.
- **Supplements**: Vitamin D3 supplements, typically in higher doses.

Calcium:

- **Cause**: Malabsorption, corticosteroid use which can decrease calcium absorption.
- **Symptoms**: Bone density loss, increased risk of osteoporosis.

Solutions:

- **Dietary Sources**: Dairy products, fortified plant-based milks, leafy green vegetables.
- **Supplements**: Calcium carbonate or calcium citrate supplements.

Folate (Vitamin B9):

- **Cause**: Malabsorption, use of certain medications like methotrexate.
- **Symptoms**: Anemia, fatigue, mouth sores.

Solutions:

- **Dietary Sources**: Leafy green vegetables, legumes, fortified cereals.
- **Supplements**: Folic acid supplements.

Magnesium:

- **Cause**: Chronic diarrhea, malabsorption.
- **Symptoms**: Muscle cramps, weakness, irregular heartbeat.

Solutions:

- **Dietary Sources**: Nuts, seeds, whole grains, green leafy vegetables.
- **Supplements**: Oral magnesium supplements.

Zinc:

- **Cause**: Chronic diarrhea, malabsorption.
- **Symptoms**: Hair loss, poor wound healing, weakened immune response.

Solutions:

- **Dietary Sources**: Meat, shellfish, legumes, seeds.
- **Supplements**: Zinc gluconate or zinc sulfate supplements.

Vitamin K:

- **Cause**: Malabsorption, particularly if fat absorption is impaired.
- **Symptoms**: Easy bruising, excessive bleeding.

Solutions:

- **Dietary Sources**: Leafy green vegetables, broccoli, Brussels sprouts.

- **Supplements**: Vitamin K1 (phylloquinone) supplements.

Additional Recommendations:

- **Regular Monitoring**: Regular blood tests to monitor nutrient levels and adjust supplementation as needed.
- **Dietitian Consultation**: Work with a registered dietitian to develop a balanced diet plan that accommodates individual needs and tolerances.
- **Enteral Nutrition**: In severe cases, particularly during flare-ups, liquid nutrition (enteral nutrition) may be necessary to ensure adequate nutrient intake while reducing bowel irritation.
- **Parenteral Nutrition**: For those who cannot absorb nutrients through their digestive tract, intravenous nutrition (parenteral nutrition) may be required.

Addressing nutritional deficiencies in Crohn's disease is crucial for managing symptoms, promoting healing, and maintaining overall health. Through a combination of dietary adjustments, supplements, and professional guidance, individuals with Crohn's disease can effectively manage these deficiencies. Regular medical monitoring and personalized nutrition plans are essential for optimal management.

CHAPTER THREE
Diet During Flares & Diet During Remission

Managing diet during flares and remission is crucial for individuals with Crohn's disease. Here are dietary recommendations for both phases:

Diet During Flares:

When experiencing a flare-up, the goal is to minimize symptoms, reduce inflammation, and prevent further irritation of the gastrointestinal tract. A diet that is gentle on the digestive system is essential.

Foods to Include:

Low-Residue, Low-Fiber Foods:

- White bread and refined pasta
- White rice
- Cooked, peeled fruits (e.g., applesauce, canned peaches)

- Cooked vegetables without skins or seeds (e.g., carrots, potatoes)

Lean Proteins:

- Skinless chicken
- Turkey
- Fish
- Eggs
- Tofu

Dairy Alternatives:

- Lactose-free milk
- Yogurt (if tolerated, especially lactose-free varieties)
- Plant-based milks (e.g., almond milk, soy milk)

Hydration:

Water:

- Herbal teas (e.g., chamomile, peppermint)

- Broths (clear, low-fat)

Easily Digestible Foods:

- Smooth nut butters (in small quantities)
- Plain cereals (e.g., Cream of Wheat)
- Mashed potatoes (without skins)
- Foods to Avoid

High-Fiber Foods:

- Whole grains
- Raw fruits and vegetables, especially those with skins or seeds
- Nuts and seeds

Fatty and Fried Foods:

- Fried foods (e.g., french fries, fried chicken)
- High-fat meats (e.g., bacon, sausage)

Spicy Foods:

- Hot peppers
- Spicy sauces and seasonings

Caffeinated and Carbonated Beverages:

- Coffee
- Tea
- Soda

Alcohol:

- Beer
- Wine
- Spirits

Sugary Foods:

- Candy
- Cakes and pastries

High-Fiber Legumes:

- Beans
- Lentils
- Chickpeas

Diet During Remission:

- When in remission, the focus shifts to maintaining nutritional balance, preventing nutrient deficiencies, and supporting overall health while avoiding known trigger foods.

Foods to Include

Balanced Diet:

- Whole grains (e.g., brown rice, quinoa, whole wheat bread)
- A variety of fruits and vegetables (cooked or raw as tolerated)
- Lean proteins (e.g., chicken, turkey, fish, eggs, tofu)

Healthy Fats:

- Olive oil
- Avocado
- Nuts and seeds (as tolerated)

Dairy and Alternatives:

- Yogurt with live cultures (probiotic varieties)
- Lactose-free dairy or plant-based alternatives

Hydration:

- Plenty of water
- Herbal teas
- Diluted fruit juices

Probiotic and Prebiotic Foods:

- Yogurt with live cultures
- Sauerkraut
- Kimchi
- Prebiotic-rich foods (e.g., garlic, onions, bananas, asparagus)

Nutrient-Rich Foods:

- Leafy green vegetables
- Fortified cereals
- Lean meats and fish
- Foods to Avoid or Limit

Known Trigger Foods:

- High-fat and fried foods
- Spicy foods
- Caffeine

- Alcohol
- High-fiber foods (if previously problematic)

Processed and Sugary Foods:

- Processed snacks (e.g., chips, cookies)
- Sugary beverages and desserts

Additional Tips

- **Keep a Food Diary**: Track foods and symptoms to identify individual triggers and tolerances.
- **Small, Frequent Meals**: Eating smaller, more frequent meals can be easier on the digestive system.
- **Chew Thoroughly**: Chewing food thoroughly can aid in digestion and reduce the risk of irritation.
- **Consult with a Dietitian**: Working with a registered dietitian can help

tailor a diet plan to individual needs and ensure nutritional adequacy.

Diet management during flares and remission is essential for individuals with Crohn's disease. During flares, focus on easily digestible, low-residue foods to minimize symptoms. In remission, aim for a balanced diet that supports overall health and prevents nutrient deficiencies while avoiding known triggers.

Personalized nutrition plans and regular consultations with healthcare providers can help optimize dietary strategies for managing Crohn's disease.

Post-Surgery Diet

After surgery for Crohn's disease, it's essential to follow a specific diet to support healing, reduce symptoms, and prevent complications. The post-surgery diet typically progresses through stages, starting with very gentle, easily digestible foods and gradually reintroducing more variety as tolerated. Here's a general guide to a post-surgery diet for Crohn's disease:

Immediate Post-Surgery Diet

1. Clear Liquid Diet

- Initially, a clear liquid diet helps ensure hydration and provides minimal stress on the digestive system.

Includes:

- Water
- Broth (clear, low-fat)

- Gelatin (without added fruit or toppings)
- Clear juices (e.g., apple, cranberry; avoid citrus)
- Herbal teas (without caffeine)

Avoid:

- Carbonated beverages
- Alcohol
- Caffeinated beverages

2. Full Liquid Diet

- As tolerance improves, the diet can advance to include more substantial liquids.

Includes:

- Milk (if tolerated, consider lactose-free options)
- Cream soups (strained, low-fat)
- Pudding and custard

- Smoothies (avoid seeds and fibrous fruits)
- Protein shakes
- Nutritional supplements (e.g., Ensure, Boost)
- Transition to Solid Foods

3. Soft Diet

- Once liquids are well-tolerated, soft, low-fiber foods can be introduced.

Includes:

- White bread, white rice, and refined pasta
- Mashed potatoes (without skins)
- Scrambled eggs
- Tender, well-cooked vegetables (without skins or seeds)
- Soft fruits (e.g., bananas, applesauce, canned peaches)

- Lean, tender meats (chicken, turkey, fish)

Avoid:

- Raw vegetables
- Whole grains
- Nuts and seeds
- Fibrous fruits (e.g., oranges, berries)

4. Low-Residue Diet:

- A low-residue diet helps to reduce bowel movements and ease the digestive process.

Includes:

- Refined grains (e.g., white bread, plain crackers)
- Cooked vegetables (carrots, green beans, peeled potatoes)
- Ripe, soft fruits (bananas, melons)

- Lean proteins (skinless chicken, fish, tofu)
- Smooth nut butters (in small amounts)
- Dairy products (if tolerated, consider lactose-free options)

Avoid:

- High-fiber vegetables (e.g., broccoli, cauliflower)
- Raw fruits with skins and seeds
- Legumes (beans, lentils)
- Spicy, fatty, and fried foods
- Gradual Reintroduction

5. Reintroduction of Regular Foods:

Slowly reintroduce a broader range of foods while monitoring tolerance and symptoms.

Steps:

- **Introduce one new food at a time**: This helps identify any food intolerances or triggers.
- **Monitor portion sizes**: Start with small portions to gauge tolerance.
- **Keep a food diary**: Track foods and symptoms to identify potential triggers.

General Tips for Post-Surgery Diet

- **Stay Hydrated**: Ensure adequate fluid intake to prevent dehydration.
- **Small, Frequent Meals**: Eat smaller, more frequent meals rather than large meals to reduce digestive stress.
- **Chew Thoroughly**: Chewing food thoroughly can aid in digestion and reduce the risk of irritation.
- **Avoid Problematic Foods**: Foods that were problematic before surgery may continue to be so; avoid them initially.

The post-surgery diet for Crohn's disease should progress gradually, starting with clear liquids and moving toward more substantial, easily digestible foods as tolerated. The key is to support healing, maintain nutrition, and prevent complications. A personalized approach, guided by healthcare providers, is essential for optimizing recovery and managing Crohn's disease effectively.

CHAPTER FOUR
Steps To Implement An Elimination Diet

Implementing an elimination diet can be a systematic process aimed at identifying specific foods that may trigger symptoms or exacerbate conditions like Crohn's disease. Here are steps to effectively implement an elimination diet:

1. Consultation with Healthcare Provider:

- Before starting an elimination diet, it's crucial to consult with a healthcare provider, preferably a registered dietitian or gastroenterologist. They can help assess your specific situation, determine if an elimination diet is appropriate, and provide guidance tailored to your health needs.

2. Define Goals and Plan:

- **Identify Symptoms**: Clearly define the symptoms or conditions you're hoping to address through the elimination diet (e.g., gastrointestinal symptoms, skin issues, fatigue).

- **Set Goals**: Determine what you aim to achieve—whether it's identifying trigger foods, improving symptoms, or achieving better overall health.

3. Choose Elimination Period:

- **Select Elimination Duration**: Typically, elimination diets involve removing potential trigger foods for a set period, often 2 to 6 weeks.

- **Gradual Approach**: Depending on the severity of symptoms and your health condition, you may opt for a gradual elimination (e.g., eliminating one food group at a time) or a comprehensive elimination of multiple potential triggers.

4. Identify Foods to Eliminate:

- **Potential Trigger Foods**: Work with your healthcare provider to identify common trigger foods based on your symptoms and medical history.

- **Common Triggers**: These may include dairy, gluten, eggs, soy, certain fruits and vegetables, nuts, and specific additives or preservatives.

5. Plan Balanced Alternative Diet:

- **Nutritional Adequacy**: Ensure your elimination diet plan includes adequate nutrients. Plan alternative foods to replace eliminated items.

- **Variety**: Include a variety of foods to prevent nutrient deficiencies and maintain interest in the diet.

6. Start Elimination Phase:

- **Clear Guidelines**: Follow clear guidelines on which foods to eliminate. Read labels carefully and avoid cross-contamination.

- **Food Diary**: Keep a detailed food diary to track everything you eat and any symptoms experienced. Note the date, time, foods consumed, and any reactions.

7. Monitor Symptoms:

- **Track Changes**: Monitor changes in symptoms throughout the elimination phase. Note any improvements or exacerbations.

- **Reactions**: Be vigilant for delayed reactions that may occur days after reintroducing eliminated foods.

8. Reintroduction Phase:

- **Systematic Reintroduction**: After the elimination phase, systematically reintroduce one eliminated food group at a time, usually every 3-5 days.

- **Observation**: Monitor symptoms closely during the reintroduction phase. If symptoms reappear, it may indicate that the reintroduced food is a trigger.

9. Evaluation and Analysis:

- **Review Results**: Evaluate the impact of each reintroduced food on symptoms.

Compare reactions to identify specific trigger foods.

- **Consultation**: Discuss findings with your healthcare provider to interpret results accurately and plan future dietary adjustments.

10. Long-Term Management:

- **Personalized Diet Plan**: Develop a personalized diet plan based on identified trigger foods and your nutritional needs.

- **Lifestyle Changes**: Incorporate long-term dietary changes to manage symptoms effectively and maintain overall health.

Tips for Success:

- **Patience and Persistence**: It may take time and multiple cycles to identify all trigger foods accurately.

- **Professional Guidance**: Seek guidance from healthcare professionals throughout the process to ensure safety and effectiveness.

- **Mindful Eating**: Pay attention to how you feel after eating and listen to your body's responses.

By following these steps and working closely with your healthcare team, you can effectively implement an elimination diet to identify trigger foods and improve your health outcomes, particularly in managing conditions like Crohn's disease.

Meal Planning For Crohn's Disease

Meal planning for Crohn's disease involves creating a balanced diet that supports digestive health, minimizes symptoms during flare-ups, and promotes overall well-being. Here's a guide to meal planning for Crohn's disease:

Principles of Meal Planning:

Balanced Nutrition

- Include a variety of foods to ensure adequate intake of nutrients.
- Focus on whole foods that are nutrient-dense and easy to digest.

Small, Frequent Meals:

- Eating smaller meals throughout the day can be easier on the digestive system.
- Aim for 5-6 smaller meals rather than 3 larger meals.

Hydration:

- Drink plenty of fluids, especially water, to stay hydrated.
- Limit or avoid caffeinated and carbonated beverages.

Consideration of Trigger Foods:

- Identify and avoid foods that trigger symptoms or exacerbate flare-ups.
- Keep a food diary to track triggers and reactions.

Meal Planning Tips:

1. Choose Easily Digestible Foods:

- **Proteins**: Lean meats (e.g., chicken, turkey), fish, eggs, tofu.
- **Carbohydrates**: White rice, refined pasta, oatmeal (if tolerated).
- **Fruits and Vegetables**: Cooked or canned fruits (without skins or seeds), well-cooked vegetables (e.g., carrots, zucchini), bananas, applesauce.

2. Meal Ideas:

Breakfast:

- Smoothies with lactose-free yogurt, banana, and almond milk.
- Oatmeal made with water or lactose-free milk, topped with a spoonful of nut butter.
- Scrambled eggs with spinach and soft cheese (if tolerated).

Lunch:

- Grilled chicken breast with white rice and steamed carrots.
- Quinoa salad with cooked vegetables (e.g., bell peppers, cucumber) and olive oil dressing.
- Tuna salad made with canned tuna, mayo (or avocado), and chopped boiled eggs, served on white bread or crackers.

Dinner:

- Baked salmon with mashed potatoes (without skins) and steamed green beans.
- Stir-fried tofu with rice noodles and cooked bell peppers in a ginger soy sauce.
- Turkey meatballs with tomato sauce served over white pasta.

Snacks:

- Rice cakes with peanut butter and sliced banana.
- Low-fat yogurt with a spoonful of honey or maple syrup.
- Cottage cheese with canned peaches (in juice, not syrup).

3. Be Mindful of Fiber:

- During flare-ups, opt for low-fiber foods such as peeled and cooked fruits and vegetables.
- Gradually introduce fiber-rich foods during remission to support gut health, but monitor tolerance.

4. Include Probiotic Foods (if tolerated):

- Yogurt with live active cultures.
- Fermented foods like sauerkraut, kimchi, or kombucha (introduce gradually).

5. Stay Organized:

- Plan meals ahead of time and prepare ingredients in advance when possible.
- Use a meal planner or app to track meals, ingredients, and symptoms.

Work with a registered dietitian who specializes in gastrointestinal health to create a personalized meal plan. They can provide guidance on specific dietary needs, supplementation, and adjustments based on individual responses.

Meal planning for Crohn's disease involves thoughtful selection of foods that support digestive health, minimize symptoms, and ensure adequate nutrition. By focusing on easily digestible, nutrient-dense foods and monitoring triggers, individuals can manage their condition effectively and improve their quality of life. Regular communication with healthcare providers and adjustments to the meal plan based on individual responses are essential for long-term management.

CHAPTER FIVE
Recipes For Easy Digestion

Here are some recipes designed to be easy on digestion, which can be beneficial for individuals managing conditions like Crohn's disease or other gastrointestinal issues. These recipes focus on using gentle ingredients that are typically well-tolerated and easy to digest:

1. Chicken and Rice Soup

Ingredients:

- 1 tablespoon olive oil
- 1 pound boneless, skinless chicken breasts, diced
- 1 onion, chopped
- 2 carrots, peeled and diced
- 2 celery stalks, diced
- 1 cup white rice, rinsed
- 6 cups low-sodium chicken broth
- Salt and pepper to taste

- Fresh parsley, chopped (optional, for garnish)

Instructions:

- In a large pot, heat olive oil over medium heat. Add diced chicken and cook until lightly browned, about 5 minutes.
- Add chopped onion, carrots, and celery to the pot. Cook, stirring occasionally, until vegetables begin to soften, about 5-7 minutes.
- Stir in rinsed white rice and chicken broth. Bring to a boil, then reduce heat to low. Cover and simmer until rice is tender and flavors are blended, about 20-25 minutes.
- Season with salt and pepper to taste. Serve hot, garnished with chopped parsley if desired.

2. Baked Salmon with Mashed Potatoes:

Ingredients:

- 4 salmon fillets (about 6 ounces each)
- 2 tablespoons olive oil
- Salt and pepper to taste
- 4 large potatoes, peeled and cubed
- 1/4 cup unsalted butter
- 1/4 cup milk (or lactose-free milk)
- Fresh dill (optional, for garnish)

Instructions:

- Preheat oven to 400°F (200°C). Place salmon fillets on a baking sheet lined with parchment paper.
- Drizzle salmon fillets with olive oil and season with salt and pepper. Bake in the preheated oven for 15-20 minutes, or until salmon flakes easily with a fork.
- While the salmon is baking, bring a large pot of water to a boil. Add cubed

potatoes and cook until tender, about 15 minutes. Drain well.
- Mash cooked potatoes with butter and milk until smooth and creamy. Season with salt and pepper to taste.
- Serve baked salmon over a bed of mashed potatoes. Garnish with fresh dill if desired.

3. Banana Oatmeal Smoothie

Ingredients:

- 1 ripe banana
- 1/2 cup rolled oats
- 1 cup lactose-free yogurt (or almond milk for dairy-free option)
- 1 tablespoon honey or maple syrup (optional, for sweetness)
- 1/2 teaspoon vanilla extract
- Ice cubes (optional, for thickness)

Instructions:

- Place all ingredients in a blender.
- Blend until smooth and creamy.
- Taste and adjust sweetness if needed by adding honey or maple syrup.
- Pour into glasses and serve immediately.

4. Turkey and Rice Stuffed Bell Peppers

Ingredients:

- 4 large bell peppers (any color)
- 1 tablespoon olive oil
- 1 pound ground turkey
- 1 onion, chopped
- 1 clove garlic, minced
- 1 cup cooked white rice
- 1 cup tomato sauce
- Salt and pepper to taste
- Fresh parsley, chopped (optional, for garnish)

Instructions:

- Preheat oven to 350°F (175°C). Cut the tops off the bell peppers and remove seeds and membranes. Place peppers upright in a baking dish.
- In a large skillet, heat olive oil over medium heat. Add ground turkey, chopped onion, and minced garlic. Cook until turkey is browned and onion is softened, about 5-7 minutes.
- Stir in cooked white rice and tomato sauce. Season with salt and pepper to taste. Cook for another 2-3 minutes to heat through.
- Spoon turkey and rice mixture evenly into each bell pepper. Cover the baking dish with foil and bake in the preheated oven for 30-35 minutes, or until peppers are tender.
- Remove from oven and garnish with chopped parsley before serving.

5. Applesauce and Cinnamon Rice Pudding:

Ingredients:

- 1 cup white rice, rinsed
- 2 cups water
- 2 cups lactose-free milk (or almond milk for dairy-free option)
- 1/2 cup unsweetened applesauce
- 1/4 cup honey or maple syrup (adjust to taste)
- 1 teaspoon ground cinnamon
- 1 teaspoon vanilla extract
- Pinch of salt
- Raisins or chopped nuts (optional, for garnish)

Instructions:

- In a medium saucepan, bring water to a boil. Add rinsed rice and reduce heat to low. Cover and simmer until rice is tender and water is absorbed, about 15-20 minutes.

- Stir in lactose-free milk, applesauce, honey or maple syrup, ground cinnamon, vanilla extract, and a pinch of salt. Cook over medium-low heat, stirring occasionally, until mixture thickens and rice is creamy, about 15-20 minutes.
- Remove from heat and let cool slightly. Serve warm or chilled, garnished with raisins or chopped nuts if desired.

Tips for Easy Digestion:

- **Cooking Methods**: Opt for gentle cooking methods like baking, steaming, or simmering.
- **Fiber**: Start with low-fiber options and gradually introduce more fiber as tolerated.
- **Portion Sizes**: Eat smaller portions to reduce digestive workload.

- **Hydration**: Drink plenty of fluids throughout the day, especially water.

These recipes provide nutritious options that are generally well-tolerated and easy on digestion, making them suitable for individuals managing Crohn's disease or other gastrointestinal conditions. Adjust ingredients based on personal tolerances and preferences, and consult with a healthcare provider or dietitian for personalized dietary advice.

7-Day Sample Meal Plan For Remission

Creating a 7-day sample meal plan for remission in Crohn's disease involves choosing foods that are gentle on the digestive system, balanced in nutrients, and avoid common trigger foods. Here's a suggested meal plan:

Day 1:

Breakfast: Banana Oatmeal Smoothie:

- Ingredients: 1 ripe banana, 1/2 cup rolled oats, 1 cup lactose-free yogurt (or almond milk), 1 tbsp honey or maple syrup, 1/2 tsp vanilla extract.

Instructions: Blend all ingredients until smooth.

Lunch: Grilled Chicken Salad:

- Grilled chicken breast over mixed greens with cucumber, cherry tomatoes, and a light vinaigrette dressing.

Dinner: Baked Salmon with Mashed Potatoes

- Baked salmon fillet with olive oil, served with mashed potatoes (made with lactose-free milk and butter).

Snack: Rice cakes with smooth peanut butter.

Day 2:

Breakfast: Scrambled Eggs with Spinach

• Scrambled eggs with cooked spinach and a slice of white toast.

Lunch: Quinoa and Vegetable Stir-Fry:

• Quinoa cooked with mixed vegetables (bell peppers, zucchini, carrots) in a light soy sauce.

Dinner: Turkey Meatballs with Tomato Sauce

• Turkey meatballs served with white rice and steamed green beans.

Snack: Low-fat yogurt with a spoonful of honey.

Day 3:

Breakfast: Smoothie Bowl:

• Smoothie bowl topped with blended berries, sliced banana, and a sprinkle of granola.

Lunch: Tuna Salad Wrap:

- Tuna salad (canned tuna, mayo or avocado, diced celery) in a whole grain tortilla wrap.

Dinner: Chicken and Rice Soup:

- Homemade chicken and rice soup with carrots, celery, and low-sodium chicken broth.

Snack: Sliced apples with smooth almond butter.

Day 4:

Breakfast: Cottage Cheese with Pineapple:

- Low-fat cottage cheese topped with fresh pineapple chunks.

Lunch: Lentil Soup:

- Homemade lentil soup with carrots, tomatoes, and spinach.

Dinner: Grilled Chicken with Quinoa Salad:

- Grilled chicken breast served with quinoa salad (quinoa, cucumber, cherry tomatoes, olive oil dressing).

Snack: Rice pudding made with lactose-free milk and topped with cinnamon.

Day 5:

Breakfast: Greek Yogurt Parfait:

- Lactose-free Greek yogurt layered with sliced strawberries and a sprinkle of granola.

Lunch: Shrimp Stir-Fry:

- Stir-fried shrimp with bell peppers, broccoli, and snap peas in a light teriyaki sauce, served over white rice.

Dinner: Baked Cod with Steamed Vegetables:

- Baked cod fillet with lemon and herbs, served with steamed carrots and green beans.

Snack: Smoothie made with almond milk, spinach, and a scoop of protein powder.

Day 6:

Breakfast: Chia Seed Pudding

- Chia seeds soaked in lactose-free milk overnight, topped with sliced bananas and a drizzle of honey.

Lunch: Chicken Caesar Salad:

- Grilled chicken breast over romaine lettuce with Caesar dressing (made with lactose-free ingredients).

Dinner: Pork Tenderloin with Roasted Potatoes:

- Roasted pork tenderloin with garlic and rosemary, served with roasted baby potatoes.

Snack: Carrot sticks with hummus.

Day 7:

Breakfast: Smoothie with Spinach and Berries

• Smoothie with almond milk, spinach, mixed berries, and a scoop of protein powder.

Lunch: Eggplant Parmesan:

• Baked eggplant slices layered with marinara sauce and mozzarella cheese, served with a side salad.

Dinner: Beef Stir-Fry with Rice Noodles:

• Stir-fried beef strips with bell peppers and broccoli in a light ginger soy sauce, served over rice noodles.

Snack: Greek yogurt with a sprinkle of granola.

Tips for Managing Crohn's Disease During Remission:

- **Hydration**: Drink plenty of water throughout the day.

- **Fiber**: Gradually introduce fiber-rich foods to support gut health.
- **Portion Sizes**: Eat smaller meals and snacks to avoid overwhelming the digestive system.
- **Monitor Symptoms**: Keep a food diary to track any reactions or symptoms.
- **Consult with a Dietitian**: Work with a registered dietitian to customize your meal plan based on individual needs and preferences.

This sample meal plan provides a variety of nutritious and easy-to-digest foods suitable for individuals in remission from Crohn's disease.

CHAPTER SIX
7-Day Sample Meal Plan For Flare-Ups

During flare-ups of Crohn's disease, it's important to focus on soothing and easily digestible foods that minimize inflammation and discomfort. Here's a sample 7-day meal plan designed to be gentle on the digestive system:

Day 1:

Breakfast:

- Smoothie with banana, lactose-free yogurt, and a spoonful of honey.

Lunch:

- White rice with boiled carrots and shredded chicken breast.

Dinner:

- Mashed potatoes with baked, skinless chicken thighs.

Snack:

- Rice cakes with smooth almond butter.

Day 2:

Breakfast:

- Scrambled eggs with well-cooked spinach.

Lunch:

- Vegetable broth soup with soft-cooked white fish.

Dinner:

- Quinoa cooked with low-sodium chicken broth and steamed zucchini.

Snack:

- Low-fat cottage cheese with sliced peaches.

Day 3

Breakfast:

- Oatmeal made with water and topped with mashed banana.

Lunch:

- Steamed white rice with boiled, peeled sweet potatoes and tofu.

Dinner:

- Baked cod fillet with steamed carrots and green beans.

Snack:

- Smoothie with lactose-free milk, strawberries, and a scoop of protein powder.

Day 4

Breakfast:

- Greek yogurt with a drizzle of honey and sliced ripe banana.

Lunch:

- Chicken and rice soup (homemade with low-fat chicken broth).

Dinner:

• Baked chicken breast with mashed butternut squash.

Snack:

• Applesauce with a sprinkle of cinnamon.

Day 5

Breakfast:

• Smoothie bowl with blended berries, almond milk, and oats.

Lunch:

• Low-residue pasta with olive oil, cooked spinach, and grilled chicken.

Dinner:

- Turkey meatballs (baked) with soft-cooked white rice and steamed broccoli.

Snack:

- Rice pudding made with lactose-free milk and topped with sliced almonds.

Day 6:

Breakfast:

- Chia seed pudding made with lactose-free milk and topped with mashed raspberries.

Lunch:

- Tuna salad (canned tuna in water, mixed with mayo or mashed avocado) on white toast.

Dinner:

- Baked salmon fillet with mashed potatoes (without skins) and boiled asparagus.

Snack:

- Smoothie with almond milk, spinach, and a tablespoon of peanut butter.

Day 7:

Breakfast:

- Cottage cheese with diced pineapple.

Lunch:

- Lentil soup (homemade with well-cooked lentils and peeled carrots).

Dinner:

- Grilled chicken breast with white rice and steamed green beans.

Snack:

- Carrot sticks with hummus.

Tips for Managing Flare-Ups

- **Hydration:** Drink plenty of water throughout the day.
- **Fiber:** Opt for low-fiber foods to reduce intestinal irritation.
- **Portion Sizes:** Eat smaller, more frequent meals to ease digestion.
- **Monitor Symptoms:** Keep a food diary to track any reactions or symptoms.
- **Consult with a Dietitian:** Work with a registered dietitian to customize your meal plan based on individual needs and preferences.

This meal plan provides a variety of nutritious and soothing foods suitable for individuals experiencing flare-ups of Crohn's disease. Adjust portions and ingredients based on personal tolerance and consult with healthcare professionals for personalized dietary guidance.

Breakfast, Lunch, And Dinner Recipes

Here are some easy-to-prepare recipes suitable for breakfast, lunch, and dinner, focusing on gentle and nutritious options that can be beneficial for individuals managing Crohn's disease:

Breakfast Recipes:

1. Banana Oatmeal Smoothie:

Ingredients:

- 1 ripe banana
- 1/2 cup rolled oats
- 1 cup lactose-free yogurt (or almond milk for dairy-free option)
- 1 tablespoon honey or maple syrup (optional, for sweetness)
- 1/2 teaspoon vanilla extract
- Ice cubes (optional, for thickness)

Instructions:

- Place all ingredients in a blender.
- Blend until smooth and creamy.
- Taste and adjust sweetness if needed by adding honey or maple syrup.
- Pour into glasses and serve immediately.

2. Scrambled Eggs with Spinach:

Ingredients:

- 2 eggs
- 1/2 cup fresh spinach, chopped
- Salt and pepper to taste
- 1 teaspoon olive oil or butter

Instructions:

- In a bowl, whisk eggs until well combined.
- Heat olive oil or butter in a non-stick skillet over medium heat.
- Add chopped spinach and cook until wilted.

- Pour in whisked eggs, stirring gently until eggs are fully cooked.
- Season with salt and pepper to taste.
- Serve hot.

Lunch Recipes:

1. Chicken and Rice Soup:

Ingredients:

- 1 tablespoon olive oil
- 1 pound boneless, skinless chicken breasts, diced
- 1 onion, chopped
- 2 carrots, peeled and diced
- 2 celery stalks, diced
- 1 cup white rice, rinsed
- 6 cups low-sodium chicken broth
- Salt and pepper to taste
- Fresh parsley, chopped (optional, for garnish)

Instructions:

- In a large pot, heat olive oil over medium heat. Add diced chicken and cook until lightly browned, about 5 minutes.
- Add chopped onion, carrots, and celery to the pot. Cook, stirring occasionally, until vegetables begin to soften, about 5-7 minutes.
- Stir in rinsed white rice and chicken broth. Bring to a boil, then reduce heat to low. Cover and simmer until rice is tender and flavors are blended, about 20-25 minutes.
- Season with salt and pepper to taste. Serve hot, garnished with chopped parsley if desired.

2. Quinoa and Vegetable Stir-Fry:

Ingredients:

- 1 cup quinoa, rinsed

- 2 cups water or low-sodium vegetable broth
- 1 tablespoon olive oil
- 1 onion, chopped
- 1 bell pepper, diced
- 1 zucchini, diced
- 1 carrot, peeled and sliced
- Soy sauce or tamari to taste
- Salt and pepper to taste

Instructions:

- In a medium saucepan, bring water or broth to a boil. Add quinoa, reduce heat to low, cover, and simmer until liquid is absorbed and quinoa is cooked, about 15-20 minutes.
- Heat olive oil in a large skillet over medium heat. Add chopped onion and cook until translucent.
- Add diced bell pepper, zucchini, and sliced carrot to the skillet. Cook,

stirring occasionally, until vegetables are tender-crisp.
- Stir in cooked quinoa and soy sauce or tamari to taste. Season with salt and pepper as needed.
- Serve warm.

Dinner Recipes

1. Baked Salmon with Mashed Potatoes:

Ingredients:

- 4 salmon fillets (about 6 ounces each)
- 2 tablespoons olive oil
- Salt and pepper to taste
- 4 large potatoes, peeled and cubed
- 1/4 cup unsalted butter
- 1/4 cup milk (or lactose-free milk)
- Fresh dill (optional, for garnish)

Instructions:

- Preheat oven to 400°F (200°C). Place salmon fillets on a baking sheet lined with parchment paper.
- Drizzle salmon fillets with olive oil and season with salt and pepper. Bake in the preheated oven for 15-20 minutes, or until salmon flakes easily with a fork.
- While the salmon is baking, bring a large pot of water to a boil. Add cubed potatoes and cook until tender, about 15 minutes. Drain well.
- Mash cooked potatoes with butter and milk until smooth and creamy. Season with salt and pepper to taste.
- Serve baked salmon over a bed of mashed potatoes. Garnish with fresh dill if desired.

2. Turkey Meatballs with Tomato Sauce:

Ingredients:

- 1 pound ground turkey
- 1/2 cup breadcrumbs (gluten-free if needed)
- 1/4 cup grated Parmesan cheese (optional)
- 1 egg
- 1 teaspoon dried oregano
- Salt and pepper to taste
- 2 cups tomato sauce (homemade or store-bought)
- Cooked white rice or pasta (optional, for serving)

Instructions:

- Preheat oven to 400°F (200°C). Line a baking sheet with parchment paper.
- In a large bowl, combine ground turkey, breadcrumbs, Parmesan cheese (if using), egg, dried oregano, salt, and pepper. Mix until well combined.

- Shape mixture into meatballs and place them on the prepared baking sheet.
- Bake meatballs in the preheated oven for 15-20 minutes, or until cooked through and lightly browned.
- Meanwhile, heat tomato sauce in a saucepan over medium heat until warmed through.
- Serve turkey meatballs with tomato sauce, over cooked white rice or pasta if desired.

Tips for Preparation:

- **Preparation Ahead:** Prep ingredients in advance to streamline cooking during busy days.
- **Portion Control:** Eat smaller, more frequent meals to aid digestion.
- **Hydration:** Drink plenty of water throughout the day to stay hydrated.

These recipes provide a variety of options for breakfast, lunch, and dinner that are gentle on the digestive system and packed with nutrients, suitable for individuals managing Crohn's disease. Adjust ingredients and seasonings based on personal preferences and dietary needs.

CHAPTER SEVEN
Snack And Smoothie Recipes

Here are some gentle snack and smoothie recipes suitable for individuals managing Crohn's disease or sensitive digestive systems:

Snack Recipes

1. Rice Cakes with Almond Butter and Banana

Ingredients*:*

- Rice cakes
- Smooth almond butter (or any nut butter of choice)
- Ripe banana, sliced

Instructions:

- Spread almond butter evenly on rice cakes.
- Top with sliced banana.
- Serve immediately.

2. Applesauce with Cinnamon:

Ingredients:

- Unsweetened applesauce
- Ground cinnamon

Instructions:

- Sprinkle ground cinnamon over applesauce.
- Stir well to combine.
- Serve chilled or at room temperature.

3. Carrot Sticks with Hummus

Ingredients:

- Carrot sticks (peeled and cut into sticks)
- Hummus (store-bought or homemade)

Instructions:

- Dip carrot sticks into hummus.

- Enjoy as a crunchy and nutritious snack.

Smoothie Recipes

1. Berry Spinach Smoothie

Ingredients:

- 1 cup fresh spinach leaves
- 1/2 cup frozen mixed berries (such as strawberries, blueberries, raspberries)
- 1/2 banana
- 1 cup lactose-free yogurt or almond milk
- 1 tablespoon honey (optional, for sweetness)

Instructions:

- Place spinach, mixed berries, banana, yogurt or almond milk, and honey (if using) in a blender.
- Blend until smooth and creamy.

- Pour into glasses and serve immediately.

2. Tropical Mango Smoothie

Ingredients:

- 1 cup frozen mango chunks
- 1/2 cup lactose-free yogurt or coconut milk
- 1/2 cup pineapple chunks (fresh or frozen)
- 1/2 banana
- 1 tablespoon chia seeds (optional, for added fiber and omega-3)

Instructions:

- Combine mango chunks, yogurt or coconut milk, pineapple chunks, banana, and chia seeds (if using) in a blender.
- Blend until smooth and creamy.
- Pour into glasses and serve chilled.

3. Green Tea Smoothie

Ingredients:

- 1 cup brewed green tea, chilled
- 1/2 cup frozen mango chunks
- 1/2 cup spinach leaves
- 1/2 banana
- 1 tablespoon honey or maple syrup (optional, for sweetness)

Instructions:

- Brew green tea and let it cool to room temperature or chill in the refrigerator.
- In a blender, combine chilled green tea, frozen mango chunks, spinach leaves, banana, and honey or maple syrup (if using).
- Blend until smooth and creamy.
- Pour into glasses and serve immediately.

Tips for Snacks and Smoothies:

- **Portion Sizes:** Enjoy snacks in small portions to avoid overwhelming the digestive system.
- **Hydration:** Drink plenty of water alongside smoothies to stay hydrated.
- **Variety:** Experiment with different fruits and vegetables in smoothies to add variety and nutrients.
- **Personalization:** Adjust sweetness levels in smoothies by adding more or less honey or maple syrup based on preference.

These snack and smoothie recipes provide nutritious options that are gentle on the digestive system, making them suitable for individuals managing Crohn's disease or other digestive conditions. Adjust ingredients based on personal preferences and dietary needs.

Specific Carbohydrate Diet (SCD) For Crohn's Disease

The Specific Carbohydrate Diet (SCD) is a dietary approach designed to manage digestive disorders like Crohn's disease by restricting certain carbohydrates that are thought to promote bacterial overgrowth and inflammation in the gut. The SCD aims to promote the healing of the gastrointestinal tract and alleviate symptoms. Here's an overview of the principles and guidelines of the Specific Carbohydrate Diet:

Principles of the Specific Carbohydrate Diet:

• **Elimination of Complex Carbohydrates:** The diet restricts complex carbohydrates that are not easily digested, including grains, certain sugars, and most dairy products.

• **Focus on Digestible Carbohydrates:** It emphasizes easily digestible carbohydrates, primarily from fruits, vegetables, and certain nuts.

- **Avoidance of Certain Additives:** Artificial additives, preservatives, and processed foods are generally avoided.

- **Emphasis on Natural and Whole Foods:** Fresh, unprocessed foods are encouraged to support digestive health.

Foods Allowed on the Specific Carbohydrate Diet:

- **Meat and Fish:** Fresh or frozen meats without additives or sugar coatings.

- **Eggs:** Eggs are generally allowed, but check for individual tolerance.

- **Non-Starchy Vegetables:** Most fresh or frozen vegetables, excluding starchy ones like potatoes.

- **Fresh Fruits:** Most fresh fruits are allowed, excluding canned or dried fruits with added sugars.

- **Nuts and Seeds:** Certain nuts and seeds are allowed, typically those that are unsalted and raw.

- **Natural Fats:** Butter, olive oil, and certain other oils are permitted.

Foods to Avoid on the Specific Carbohydrate Diet:

- **Grains:** All grains and products made from them, including bread, pasta, and cereal.
- **Processed Foods:** Processed meats, canned goods, and foods with additives or artificial ingredients.
- **Certain Dairy Products:** Most dairy is restricted initially; some may tolerate homemade yogurt with specific bacterial strains over time.
- **Starchy Vegetables:** Potatoes, corn, and other starchy vegetables are typically avoided.
- **Certain Sweeteners:** All refined sugars, artificial sweeteners, and most natural sweeteners are avoided initially.

Sample Day on the Specific Carbohydrate Diet:

Breakfast:

- Scrambled eggs with spinach cooked in olive oil

Lunch:

- Grilled chicken breast with steamed carrots and homemade applesauce

Dinner:

- Baked salmon with a side of butternut squash puree and sautéed zucchini

Snacks:

• Fresh fruit (e.g., apple slices with almond butter)

• Homemade yogurt made from lactose-free milk or almond milk (once tolerated)

Additional Considerations:

• **Introduction Phase:** The SCD typically begins with an introductory phase where the diet is very restrictive to allow the gut to heal. Foods are gradually reintroduced based on individual tolerance.

• **Individual Variation:** The diet may need to be customized based on individual response and tolerance to specific foods.

The Specific Carbohydrate Diet can be effective for some individuals with Crohn's disease in managing symptoms and promoting gut health. However, as with any dietary approach, it's essential to seek personalized guidance and monitoring from healthcare professionals to ensure it meets individual nutritional needs and health goals.

Gluten-Free Diet For Crohn's Disease

A gluten-free diet involves eliminating gluten, a protein found in wheat, barley, rye, and sometimes oats, which can trigger inflammation and exacerbate symptoms in individuals with certain autoimmune conditions, including Crohn's disease.

Here's a guide to following a gluten-free diet for managing Crohn's disease:

Principles of a Gluten-Free Diet:

Avoidance of Gluten-Containing Grains:

- Wheat (including varieties like durum, semolina, and spelt)
- Barley
- Rye

- Some oats (due to cross-contamination; choose certified gluten-free oats)

Focus on Naturally Gluten-Free Foods:

- Fruits and vegetables
- Lean meats, poultry, and fish
- Legumes (beans and lentils)
- Nuts and seeds
- Dairy products (check for hidden gluten in flavored or processed dairy products)

Gluten-Free Grains and Alternatives:

- Rice (including brown, white, and wild rice)
- Quinoa
- Corn
- Gluten-free oats (certified gluten-free to avoid cross-contamination)
- Buckwheat

- Millet
- Amaranth
- Tapioca

Read Labels Carefully:

- Avoid processed foods that may contain hidden sources of gluten, such as sauces, dressings, soups, and processed meats.
- Look for gluten-free labels or certifications on packaged foods.

Sample Gluten-Free Meal Plan for Crohn's Disease:

Breakfast:

• Quinoa porridge made with almond milk, topped with fresh berries and a drizzle of honey

Lunch:

- Grilled chicken salad with mixed greens, cherry tomatoes, cucumber, and avocado (dressing made with olive oil and lemon juice)

Dinner:

- Baked salmon fillet with a side of gluten-free pasta (made from rice or quinoa) and steamed broccoli

Snacks:

- Rice cakes with almond butter and banana slices

- Greek yogurt with gluten-free granola

Tips for Following a Gluten-Free Diet with Crohn's Disease:

- **Cook from Scratch:** Prepare meals using whole, naturally gluten-free ingredients to better control what you eat.

- **Check for Cross-Contamination:** Be cautious when dining out or using shared kitchen utensils and equipment that may have had contact with gluten-containing foods.

- **Monitor Symptoms:** Keep a food diary to track any reactions or symptoms that may indicate gluten sensitivity or intolerance.

Following a gluten-free diet can help reduce inflammation and manage symptoms in some individuals with Crohn's disease. However, it's essential to customize the diet based on individual tolerance and seek professional guidance to ensure nutritional needs are met and health goals are achieved effectively.

Low-FODMAP Diet For Crohn's Disease

The Low-FODMAP diet is a dietary approach that restricts certain types of carbohydrates (FODMAPs) that are poorly absorbed in the small intestine and can trigger symptoms in individuals with irritable bowel syndrome (IBS) and potentially in those with Crohn's disease or other digestive disorders.

While research on the specific benefits of the Low-FODMAP diet in Crohn's disease is ongoing and individual responses vary, some people find symptom relief and improved quality of life by reducing FODMAP intake. Here's an overview of the Low-FODMAP diet and how it may be applied for Crohn's disease:

FODMAPs are short-chain carbohydrates and sugar alcohols that are fermented by gut bacteria and can cause symptoms like bloating, gas, abdominal pain, and diarrhea in sensitive individuals. The term FODMAP stands for:

- **Fermentable:** Easily fermented by gut bacteria.
- **Oligosaccharides:** Includes fructans and galacto-oligosaccharides (GOS)

found in foods like wheat, onions, garlic, and legumes.

- **Disaccharides:** Includes lactose found in dairy products.
- **Monosaccharides:** Includes excess fructose found in certain fruits and sweeteners like honey and agave syrup.
- **Polyols:** Includes sugar alcohols like sorbitol, mannitol, xylitol, and maltitol found in certain fruits, vegetables, and artificial sweeteners.

Low-FODMAP Diet Guidelines:

The Low-FODMAP diet typically involves three phases:

- **Elimination Phase:** Initially, all high-FODMAP foods are eliminated for a period of 2-6 weeks to reduce symptoms.

- **Reintroduction Phase:** High-FODMAP foods are systematically reintroduced one at a time to identify which specific FODMAPs trigger symptoms and at what threshold.
- **Personalization Phase:** Based on individual tolerance levels, a personalized long-term diet is developed that includes a variety of foods while minimizing FODMAPs that trigger symptoms.

Foods to Include on a Low-FODMAP Diet:

- **Proteins:** Meat, poultry, fish, eggs.
- **Low-FODMAP Vegetables:** Bell peppers, spinach, zucchini, carrots, cucumber, tomatoes (in moderation).
- **Fruits (in small servings):** Strawberries, blueberries, grapes, oranges, kiwi.

- **Grains:** Gluten-free grains like rice, quinoa, oats (if tolerated).
- **Dairy (lactose-free or low-lactose):** Lactose-free milk, hard cheeses (like cheddar or Swiss), lactose-free yogurt.
- **Fats:** Oils, butter, most nuts and seeds in moderation.

Foods to Avoid or Limit on a Low-FODMAP Diet:

- **High-FODMAP Vegetables:** Onions, garlic, cauliflower, broccoli, asparagus, mushrooms.
- **Fruits:** Apples, pears, cherries, watermelon, mango, dried fruits.
- **Dairy:** Milk, soft cheeses, yogurt (if not lactose-free).
- **Grains:** Wheat, rye, barley, and products made from them.

- **Sweeteners:** High-fructose corn syrup, honey, agave syrup, sorbitol, mannitol, xylitol.

Sample Low-FODMAP Meal Plan for Crohn's Disease:

Breakfast:

- Scrambled eggs with spinach and tomatoes (cooked without onion or garlic)
- Gluten-free toast with lactose-free butter

Lunch:

- Grilled chicken with quinoa salad (quinoa, cucumber, cherry tomatoes, and a drizzle of olive oil and lemon juice)

Dinner:

- Baked salmon with steamed carrots and a side of rice

Snacks:

- Strawberries with lactose-free yogurt
- Rice cakes with natural peanut butter

Tips for Following a Low-FODMAP Diet with Crohn's Disease:

- **Consultation:** Work with a registered dietitian experienced in the Low-FODMAP diet to ensure nutritional adequacy and proper implementation.

- **Personalization:** Modify the diet based on individual responses and tolerances.
- **Monitoring:** Keep a food and symptom diary to track how different foods affect symptoms and adjust accordingly.
- **Long-Term Maintenance:** Once trigger foods are identified, reintroduce tolerated foods to maintain a balanced diet and meet nutritional needs.

The Low-FODMAP diet can be a valuable tool for managing symptoms in individuals with Crohn's disease, but it should be implemented under the guidance of a healthcare professional to ensure it meets individual dietary needs and health goals.

Vegan And Vegetarian Diets For Crohn's Disease

Vegan and vegetarian diets, which exclude or minimize animal products, can be considered for managing Crohn's disease. These diets emphasize plant-based foods, which can be rich in fiber, antioxidants, and nutrients that support overall health and may aid in reducing inflammation.

However, managing Crohn's disease with a vegan or vegetarian diet requires careful planning to ensure nutritional adequacy and to minimize potential triggers. Here are some considerations and tips for adopting vegan or vegetarian diets with Crohn's disease:

Considerations for Vegan and Vegetarian Diets:

- **Fiber Content:** Plant-based diets tend to be higher in fiber, which can be beneficial for digestive health but may exacerbate symptoms during flare-ups. It's important to monitor fiber intake and choose easily digestible sources.

- **Nutrient Deficiencies:** Vegan diets, in particular, may be deficient in certain nutrients such as vitamin B12, iron, zinc, omega-3 fatty acids, and protein. Vegetarian diets may also need attention to ensure adequate iron and omega-3 intake.

- **Potential Triggers:** Some high-fiber foods (like beans, legumes, cruciferous vegetables) and certain raw fruits and vegetables may trigger symptoms such as bloating, gas, and diarrhea in individuals with Crohn's disease.

Tips for Vegan and Vegetarian Diets with Crohn's Disease:

Focus on Nutrient-Dense Foods:

- **Proteins:** Incorporate plant-based protein sources such as legumes (lentils, chickpeas), tofu, tempeh, and quinoa.

- **Iron:** Include iron-rich foods like spinach, lentils, tofu, and fortified cereals.
- **Omega-3s:** Consume sources such as ground flaxseeds, chia seeds, walnuts, and algae-based supplements.
- **B12:** Ensure adequate intake through fortified foods (like nutritional yeast and fortified plant milks) or supplements.
- **Cooking Methods:** Opt for cooking methods that are gentle on the digestive system, such as steaming, boiling, or sautéing, to make food easier to digest.
- **Monitor Fiber Intake:** During flare-ups or periods of active symptoms, choose low-fiber options such as

peeled and well-cooked vegetables, cooked fruits, and refined grains.
- **Stay Hydrated:** Drink plenty of water throughout the day to maintain hydration, especially if increasing fiber intake.
- **Experiment and Adjust:** Keep a food diary to track how different foods affect symptoms. Gradually introduce new foods and monitor reactions to identify potential triggers.

Sample Vegan and Vegetarian Meal Plan for Crohn's Disease:

Breakfast:

- Smoothie with spinach, banana, almond milk, and chia seeds
- Overnight oats made with almond milk, topped with berries and a spoonful of almond butter

Lunch:

- Quinoa salad with mixed greens, chickpeas, cucumber, cherry tomatoes, and a lemon-tahini dressing

Dinner:

- Stir-fried tofu with broccoli, bell peppers, and carrots served over brown rice

Snacks:

- Hummus with carrot sticks
- A handful of nuts (like almonds or walnuts)

Additional Tips:

- **Supplementation:** Consider supplements as needed, particularly for vitamin B12, iron, and omega-3 fatty acids. Consult with a healthcare provider or dietitian for personalized recommendations.

- **Professional Guidance:** Work with a registered dietitian experienced in vegan or vegetarian nutrition to ensure your diet meets nutritional needs and supports your health goals.
- **Balanced Approach:** Aim for a balanced diet that includes a variety of plant-based foods to maximize nutrient intake and support overall health.

Adopting a vegan or vegetarian diet with Crohn's disease can be beneficial with careful planning and monitoring. It's essential to prioritize nutrient adequacy and consider individual tolerance to different foods to manage symptoms effectively.

CHAPTER EIGHT
Lifestyle And Dietary Strategies For Long-Term Management

Managing Crohn's disease involves a multifaceted approach that goes beyond medication to include lifestyle and dietary strategies aimed at reducing inflammation, managing symptoms, and promoting overall health and well-being. Here are some key lifestyle and dietary strategies for long-term management of Crohn's disease:

Lifestyle Strategies:

Stress Management:

- Practice stress-reducing techniques such as mindfulness meditation, yoga, deep breathing exercises, or hobbies that promote relaxation.

- Prioritize adequate sleep and establish a regular sleep schedule to support overall well-being.

Regular Exercise:

• Engage in regular physical activity that is appropriate for your condition and fitness level. Exercise can help reduce inflammation, manage stress, and improve overall health.

• Choose activities that you enjoy and can sustain, such as walking, swimming, cycling, or yoga.

Smoking Cessation:

• If you smoke, quitting smoking is crucial for managing Crohn's disease. Smoking has been linked to worsening symptoms and increased disease severity.

Hydration:

• Drink plenty of water throughout the day to maintain hydration, especially if you have diarrhea or are prone to dehydration due to medication or flare-ups.

Regular Medical Follow-Up:

• Maintain regular follow-up appointments with your healthcare provider to monitor disease activity, adjust treatment as needed, and address any concerns or new symptoms promptly.

Dietary Strategies:

Personalized Diet Approach:

- Work with a registered dietitian or healthcare provider to develop a personalized diet plan that takes into account your specific symptoms, nutritional needs, and food tolerances.

- Consider diets such as the low-FODMAP diet, Specific Carbohydrate Diet (SCD), or gluten-free diet if they are found to alleviate symptoms.

Balanced Nutrition:

- Aim for a balanced diet rich in whole foods, including fruits, vegetables, lean proteins, healthy fats, and whole grains (if tolerated).

- Ensure adequate intake of essential nutrients such as vitamins (especially B12), minerals (iron and calcium), and omega-3 fatty acids.

Fiber Management:

- Monitor and adjust your fiber intake based on symptoms. During flare-ups, opt for low-fiber foods such as well-cooked vegetables, peeled fruits, and refined grains. Gradually reintroduce higher-fiber foods during remission.

Hydration and Electrolytes:

- If you experience diarrhea or dehydration, consume electrolyte-rich fluids such as sports drinks or oral rehydration solutions under the guidance of your healthcare provider.

Food Diary:

- Keep a food diary to track your diet and symptoms. This can help identify trigger foods and patterns that worsen or alleviate symptoms.

__Additional Considerations:__

- **Medication Adherence:** Take medications as prescribed by your healthcare provider to manage inflammation and control symptoms effectively.
- **Support Network:** Seek support from family, friends, or support groups for emotional and practical support in managing Crohn's disease.
- **Education:** Stay informed about Crohn's disease, treatment options, and self-management strategies. Knowledge empowers you to make informed decisions about your health.

By adopting these lifestyle and dietary strategies, you can effectively manage Crohn's disease over the long term, reduce the frequency and severity of flare-ups, and improve your overall quality of life. It's essential to work closely with your healthcare team to tailor these strategies to your individual needs and monitor your condition regularly.

Common Questions About Crohn's And Diet

Here are some common questions about Crohn's disease and diet, along with brief answers:

Can diet cure Crohn's disease?

Diet cannot cure Crohn's disease, but it can help manage symptoms and improve quality of life.

What diet is recommended for Crohn's disease?

There is no one-size-fits-all diet for Crohn's. However, a low-residue or low-fiber diet during flare-ups and a balanced, nutrient-rich diet during remission are often recommended.

Are there specific foods to avoid with Crohn's disease?

Trigger foods vary among individuals, but common ones include spicy foods, high-fiber foods, dairy products (if lactose intolerant), and certain raw fruits and vegetables.

Should I take supplements with Crohn's disease?

Supplements like iron, vitamin B12, and vitamin D may be necessary due to malabsorption issues. Consult with a healthcare provider to determine specific needs.

Is it safe to drink alcohol with Crohn's disease?

Alcohol can exacerbate symptoms and interfere with medications. It's generally recommended to limit or avoid alcohol, especially during flare-ups.

Can probiotics help with Crohn's disease?

Probiotics may benefit some people with Crohn's by promoting gut health, but their effectiveness varies. Consult with a healthcare provider before starting probiotics.

Is it okay to follow a vegetarian or vegan diet with Crohn's disease?

Vegetarian and vegan diets can be adapted for Crohn's disease, but careful planning is essential to ensure adequate nutrition and avoid potential trigger foods.

How can I manage weight with Crohn's disease?

Maintaining a healthy weight is important. If you have trouble gaining or losing weight due to Crohn's, a dietitian can help create a plan tailored to your needs.

What should I do if I have a nutrition-related question about Crohn's disease?

Consult with a registered dietitian or gastroenterologist who specializes in inflammatory bowel diseases for personalized advice.

Can stress affect Crohn's disease symptoms related to diet?

Yes, stress can exacerbate symptoms. Managing stress through relaxation techniques, exercise, and support groups may help improve overall well-being.

For information that is particular to your condition and needs, it is necessary to consult healthcare professionals. These responses provide a general overview.

Summary

Managing Crohn's disease calls for a holistic strategy that incorporates personalized food and lifestyle recommendations with medical treatment.

Adopting good lifestyle practices can greatly improve overall well-being and quality of life for those with Crohn's disease, in addition to drugs, which are essential for reducing inflammation and symptoms.

Reducing inflammation and maintaining immune function requires a change in lifestyle, which includes things like quitting smoking, getting enough sleep, exercising regularly, and managing stress. In addition to alleviating symptoms, these techniques also have positive effects on your health in the long run.

The low-FODMAP diet, the Specific Carbohydrate Diet (SCD), the gluten-free diet, and other individualized diets based on tolerance and response are some of the dietary tactics that play an important part in the management of Crohn's disease.

Important factors to optimize digestive health include maintaining a balanced nutritional intake, controlling fiber consumption, and monitoring water levels.

Being well-informed about Crohn's disease and treatment options is essential for good management, as is keeping frequent medical follow-up appointments and taking drugs as prescribed. Collaboration between gastroenterologists and registered dietitians, among other healthcare professionals, allows for the development of individualized treatment programs that may be fine-tuned as needed for the best possible results.

Better symptom control, less flare-up frequency, and improved quality of life can be achieved by incorporating these methods into everyday living and working collaboratively with healthcare experts by those with Crohn's disease. In order to effectively treat Crohn's disease over the long term, it is crucial to provide continuous support and education, as each person's path with the disease is different.

THE END

www.ingramcontent.com/pod-product-compliance
Lightning Source LLC
Chambersburg PA
CBHW071831210526
45479CB00001B/89